ADD Simplified

Strategies for Minimizing the Effects of Adult ADD and ADHD

Sidney Parker Holt

I0156660

HENDRIX INTERNATIONAL PRESS

ADD Simplified – Strategies for Minimizing the Effects of Adult ADD and ADHD (Paperback Edition)

Published by Hendrix International Press, an imprint of Hendrix International, LLC. Printed in the United States of America.

ISBN-10: 0-9831511-1-3
ISBN-13: 978-0-9831511-1-1
Library of Congress Control Number: 2010941160

The information and advice presented in this book are not meant to substitute for the advice of your physician or other trained health-care professionals. You are advised to consult with health-care professionals with regard to all matters that may require medical attention or diagnosis and to check with a physician before administering or undertaking any course of treatment or diet.

Publisher's Cataloging-in-Publication

Holt, Sidney Parker.

ADD Simplified : Strategies for minimizing the effects of Adult ADD and ADHD / Sidney Parker Holt, 1st ed. Revision #2.
p. cm.
Includes bibliographical references and index.

Classification Terms

1. Attention-Deficit Hyperactivity Disorder-Popular Works
2. Attention-Deficit Disorder in Adults-Popular Works
3. I. Holt, Sidney Parker

Hendrix International, LLC
16192 Coastal Highway,
Lewes, DE 19958
USA

Roy Dictus, Publisher – roy@hendrix-int.com

The author welcomes your feedback at sidney@addsimplified.com.

http://www.addsimplified.com

This book is dedicated to Hakim (1974-2010); trusted colleague, dear friend, ADDer, and one of the first proofreaders of this book. Hakim, nobody who ever knew you will ever forget you.

Advance Praise for ADD Simplified

"Concise tips, clearly written and presented. Sidney Parker Holt zeroes in on core strategies that work."

— Gina Pera, author, *"Is It You, Me, Or Adult A.D.D.?"*

"A great collection of tips and ideas. It's also written in a very accessible (easy to understand) style."

— Jeff Siegel, blogger, *"Jeff's ADD Mind"*

"ADD Simplified is virtually the handbook I've been dreaming of to teach my AD/HD child the skills necessary to one day be a successful AD/HD adult. It contains remarkably simple strategies for organization, planning, and time management, in small bites even the most distracted mind can handle."

— Penny Williams, blogger, *"A Mom's View of ADHD"*

CONTENTS

Introduction to the Paperback edition 7

PART 1 : KEEPING TRACK 9

Don't Leave Home Without It 11

Use Color-Coding Effectively 13

The Label Maker is your Friend 17

Checklists Help You Keep Track 21

Kanban: To-Do Lists on Steroids 23

Keep Track of Important Documents 27

PART 2: DEALING WITH CLUTTER 29

Reduce Clutter by Letting Go 31

Give Everything its Own Place 35

Reduce Visual Clutter 39

Don't Turn Your Living Room or Bedroom into Something Else 41

Filing Cabinets to the Rescue 45

Electronics for Clutter Management 49

PART 3: MONEY MATTERS 51

Budgeting to Track and Keep Your Money 53

Impulse Control when Shopping – or, "Do I *Really* Want This?" ... 55

The Low-Limit Credit Card 59

Some More Money Tips 61

PART 4: DEALING WITH PROCRASTINATION 63

I'll Do it Tomorrow 65

Penalties and Rewards 67

Don't Be Late, Now 69

The "Do It Now" Attitude 73

Electronics for Time Management 75

PART 5: REDUCING STRESS 77

Perfection Doesn't Exist – Accept "Good Enough" 79

One Thing at a Time; You're Not a Juggler 81

Avoid Morning Stress..85

Establish a Bedtime Ritual 89

Power Naps are Good for You 93

Prepare For Important Conversations............................95

Time and Attention Magnets Lead to Compulsion.........97

Build a Support System...101

BONUS SECTION: 4 x 10 105

10 Reasons to Invest in a Smartphone 107

10 Books to Read 113

10 Websites to Explore..117

10 Blogs about ADD 121

Final Thoughts 124

ADD Simplified, Other Editions.....................................125

Index 126

Introduction to the Paperback edition

This book is for adults with ADD or ADHD. I hope that it will help you eliminate some of the daily chaos that makes living with AD(H)D harder, and will help you cope with the rest.

Note that all over the book, I've used the acronym ADD in the title rather than ADHD or AD(H)D, AD/HD etc. because it is still the most common way people refer to the phenomenon.

But first, let me introduce myself. My name is Sidney and I am a 42-year-old freelance IT consultant with ADD. I have struggled with ADD all my life, and over the years I have gathered a set of strategies to help me cope with it. I decided to write them down to share them with fellow ADDers. Some of these strategies I learned from ADD "colleagues", others I came up with myself. I'm sure you'll recognize some of them, and others will be new.

The techniques I describe here come from personal experience. This book does not list the symptoms of ADD or tell you what supplements to take. There are enough books like that on the market.

Structure is the key to many of the strategies discussed in this book. As we are inherently chaotic, we need more structure than "ordinary" people to function. We need schedules, routines and anything tangible that reduces disorder.

Automation is another key principle behind the strategies. Many of our problems go away when we can automate certain processes. We will look at many ways to automatically deal with the challenges we face.

The third and final key principle is a *"Go For It!" attitude*. Once you have that – and I'm guessing you are already there, or nearly, otherwise you wouldn't be reading this – the rest becomes more manageable.

Some strategies will work for you, and others won't. It's up to you to discover which of these practical techniques will help you. Even in our ADD we are not quite all alike.

I have tried to write this book in a clear and straightforward style, easy to browse and easy to read: just the way us Attention-Deficit sufferers like it. You can start with any chapter and read the chapters in any order. They are concise, practical and to the point. The book is also available in both electronic (e-book) and paperback formats.

One last remark: a number of pages in this book are indeed blank, save for the page number. This is the result of layout. We did not write *"This page intentionally left blank"* on these pages for two very simple reasons: (1) it's annoying and (2) it's distracting.

But enough talk already, let's get on with it!

Sidney

PART 1

KEEPING TRACK

Don't Leave Home Without It

Don't you hate it when, too long after leaving the house, you suddenly remember that you forgot something important at home?

Here are some smart tactics to counter this concern:

Group items together

Chances are, you'll have to take more than one item with you when you leave. Group them together on the table: your keys, your wallet, your e-reader. What are the chances you'll forget them all?

If the table is not a good place, pick another spot that you are guaranteed to see before you leave.

Put item(s) in or on your shoes

Very likely you will not forget to put on your shoes. So put your item on or in your shoes, or put your shoes on top of your item. If you *do* tend to forget to put on your shoes, drop them right in front of the door.

In a similar fashion, when there's something you absolutely need to do before bed, you can put a little reminder on your pillow or on the bathroom mirror.

Hang it over the doorknob

Do you need to take a bag or a piece of clothing (like a scarf) with you? Hang it neatly over the doorknob so that you cannot leave without seeing and touching it.

Put it in the trunk of your car in advance

If you can, why not put the item where it needs to be when you think of it? If you live in a safe neighborhood, you may even put it on the passenger seat so that you'll see it when you get in the car in the morning.

Set a reminder alarm

For me this happens to be one of the less-potent options, as I tend to ignore reminder alarms when I'm busy (which is always). But just letting your phone or watch remind you what to do right before you leave may do the trick. One thing that helps me to attend to the alarm is when the beep is very annoying.

Keys, phone and wallet

These are generally the items you always carry with you. So give them a fixed place, so that you always know where to find them and you can quickly check whether you have them with you.

For instance, I always keep my keys in my right-front pocket and my phone in my left-front pocket. Always. When I leave the house or when I'm in the city, I regularly pat my pockets to make sure everything is still there. It may seem silly, but since I started doing that, I've never left the house without my keys. Also, if one day some handy pickpocket succeeds in stealing my phone on the street, it won't take long before I notice it's gone. Maybe it won't be too late.

Keep a mirror near your front door

If you have a mirror near your front door, you can always quickly check yourself before you leave. This is convenient and you never have to run to the bathroom for that final check, wasting precious time.

Use Color-Coding Effectively

Reading is fast, recognizing color is faster. Therefore, we can find what we're looking for a lot faster if we use color-coding. You can apply this simple principle everywhere.

Color-coding works wonders when you have to find that needle in your haystack – any haystack!

Color-code keys

For example, you can buy colored rings to slide around your keys: for instance, the red ring for your front-door key, the yellow ring for the office key. You can also get colored keys.

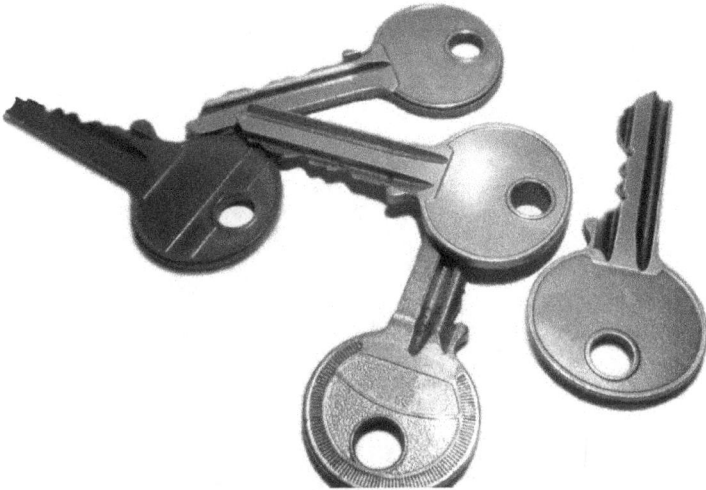

Persuade everyone in your family to color-code their keys if you have to. This is helpful for everyone, ADD or no, and you can easily find the right key when you have to get in with your partner's set.

Drawers and folders

When you label drawers, you can get colored label tape to categorize them. For instance, blue labels for his stuff, red labels for hers; or yellow labels for purchase-related shelves, and green labels for sales-related ones.

Color-coding also works fine with folders. I use blue folders for documents related to the house, white folders for documents related to official paperwork (taxes), a green folder for all medical documents, etc.

Within a folder, you can also stick mini sticky labels to individual documents. I use these to find back important chapters in reference manuals.

In the house, at the office

In our living room, we have an Ikea filing cabinet with square open sections. Ikea also sells fabric boxes you can use as drawers in this cabinet. And, as luck would have it, they sell these in multiple colors. So we put the kids' toys in the blue boxes/drawers and mom's stuff in the black ones.

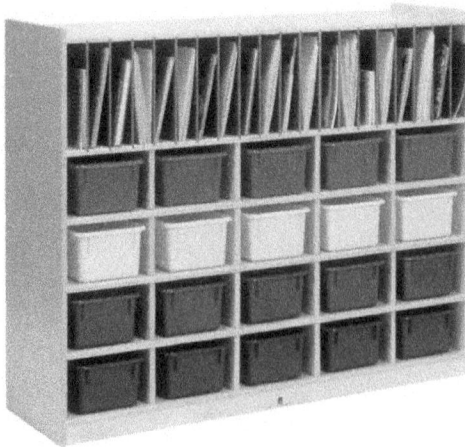

E-mail

How about e-mail? Advanced programs such as Outlook and Gmail support color-coding incoming mails. You can easily set up rules to automatically apply labels and color codes. For instance, you may instruct your e-mail program to color-code a mail sent directly to you by your boss, and mark it *Urgent* in red. Those mails then stand out in the list of received messages. Likewise, messages coming from important customers, your family, etc., can each be color-coded differently. This way, you can reduce the time you need to spend scanning e-mails to find the important ones, almost without effort.

Luggage

When you travel, use luggage that catches the eye. If you have a fluorescent yellow-and-green suitcase with a big *I Love Mashed Potatoes* sticker on it, it's unlikely that someone else will walk away with it. And will you accidentally take home someone else's gear? This, too, is a way of color-coding.

Don't use more than five colors

The benefits of color-coding go away once you use more than five colors. It just becomes too difficult for most of us to keep track of the meaning of each color. So stick to a selection of up to five colors and use them consistently.

Think of ways you can apply color-coding in your life to make finding things easier.

The Label Maker is your Friend

An electronic label maker is a must-have. Labeling boxes, bags, drawers, computer supplies, medications etc. simplifies things radically. Labeled items are so much neater, more organized and easier to find back, and labeling takes almost no effort.

Get a flexible label maker

My personal label maker has a keyboard and a rechargeable battery. These can print on a variety of labels: white or colored, paper or plastic, wide or narrow; and in a variety of fonts and weights: standard, bold, slanted, etc. Such labelers are a bit more expensive than average labelers, but they're worth it. The flexibility you get with these devices makes labeling easier and much more fun.

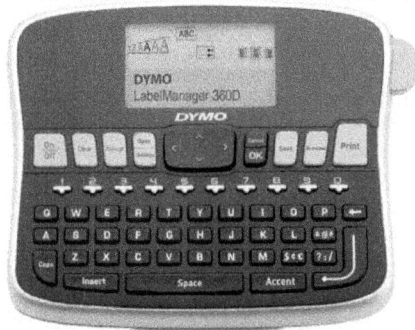

Here are some examples where a label maker can make a difference:

Meds

Say you have a medicine cabinet full of bottles and you quickly need an antacid. If your meds are marked with big bold labels, finding the right bottle (and not accidentally taking out the wrong one) becomes a piece of cake. You may also want to print the dosage on the label if it is the same for everyone in the household, or mark dosage information with a magic marker.

Food

Got a freezer full of prepared food? Get out the labeler next time you cook and mark each box with the contents and date of preparation. Use big, bold letters so that you can easily find back the right box later when you're hungry and there's frosting on the lids.

In the fridge, the labeler helps out too by quickly identifying the container that holds the light cheese. Alternatively, you may use color-coded labels to distinguish "diet" meals from heavier ones, etc.

If you are a student and you share a fridge in the dormitory with others, you may want to mark your milk too – although you won't need a labeler for that, a Sharpie will do.

In and Out Trays

If you want to get highly organized, you can use *In* and *Out* trays for every member of the family or the office. And here comes the label maker again, to mark which tray is which.

Toys

If you have kids who share a drawer chest for their toys, you may label drawers to keep similar toys together: **Danny's Robots**, **Sheila's Barbies**, and so on. This makes it so much easier for the kids to find back their toys. When a doll is missing, you know where to look and where not to look. After play, these labeled drawers again make cleaning up the room a stress-free job – everything has its own, clearly marked, destination.

Again, you can use color-coding (labels of different colors) to make finding back the right drawer a snap.

Boxes

Label your boxes with their contents: **Family Photos**, **Stamps**, etc. There's no need to be elaborate; just describe the contents in a few words, so that you can find the right box quickly.

Cables

Check out that web of tangled cables behind the TV. What cable goes where? Label those cables with **TV**, **Media Player**, **Console**, etc. *on both ends,* and you'll never pull out the wrong one any longer.

Gifts

Never accidentally hand grandpa your mom's gift again!

The possibilities are endless.

Checklists Help You Keep Track

Before any airplane takes off, its pilots have determined that everything was ready for a safe flight. They know it is because they ran a safety checklist. This checklist contains a number of conditions the pilots must check and mark. Is there enough fuel for the trip, plus some more to be able to handle route changes and a waiting line to land? Do all the engines work? What about tire pressure? All of these conditions must be checked off, or the plane is not deemed safe. Similarly, surgical teams use checklists before operations to make sure conditions for the operation are right. In fact, Dr. Atul Gawande, who came up with a checklist for heart surgery procedures, wrote his ideas and experiences down in *The Checklist Manifesto*, published by Metropolitan Books.

Now, if pilots and surgeons – not exactly people known for their goofiness or confused minds – need checklists to make sure they don't forget anything, why would we not use them?

We can use checklists for so many things. My family uses a checklist before our kids go on sleepovers, for instance:

o   Parents are expecting us at _____
o   We pick up Robin up on _____ at _____
o   The address is _____ _____
o   Parents' phone: _____
o   Contact page with our phone numbers and email addresses
o   Pajamas
o   Teddy bear
o   Toothbrush
o   Underwear + spare
o   T-shirt + spare

- o   Spare pants
- o   3 books

...

In the preparation time for the sleepover, we check each item so that we know when we're *really* ready to leave.

It's important to check any item on the list as soon as it's verified so that nobody attempts double work. Checklists remind you what you need to remember and they show progress. It's virtually impossible now to forget to pack or do anything important.

We also have a checklist for day trips, garage cleaning day, grocery shopping, etc. Anything that requires a number of steps or items to pack is a good candidate for a checklist even if you know what to do by heart. There are always days when you need to rely on the security a checklist provides. Ask any pilot or heart surgeon you know.

Whiteboard, hard copy, or smartphone?

For a quick, one-time checklist, the whiteboard is a good place to write it down. You can use a word processor or spreadsheet to draw up recurring checklists; that is, lists that you'll often use. Print out a hard copy and put it on the whiteboard with a magnet.

If the checklist is just for you, you might as well keep it on your smartphone. For all of today's smartphones, you can download commercial or free checklist applications. The one I prefer is called **Springpad** (see *http://springpadit.com*); this is both a Web application and a smartphone application, for managing quick notes (think electronic sticky notes) and checklists. Any change you make in a checklist on your phone is automatically synchronized to the Web version of that list, and vice versa. Excellent!

See also "10 Reasons to Invest in a Smartphone".

Kanban: To-Do Lists on Steroids

A very special case of the to-do list, or task checklist, is the **Kanban** system. This is a Japanese-invented tracking system that gives you an overview of what is going on and what still needs to happen (and even who is doing it). Kanban was originally invented by the car industry for just-in-time inventory control, but you can apply it everywhere – at home, at the office, at the factory, at school – and it's especially interesting for us who need help with keeping track.

So what is it? It's a system where you keep track of things to do by writing them down, say, on sticky notes (yes, there are computer-based versions of Kanban available, but let's stick with the paper version for now). You put these notes on a whiteboard, or alternatively, pin them on a cork bulletin board.

This *Kanban board* has columns on it, for instance: *Backlog, Ready, Ongoing* and *Done*.

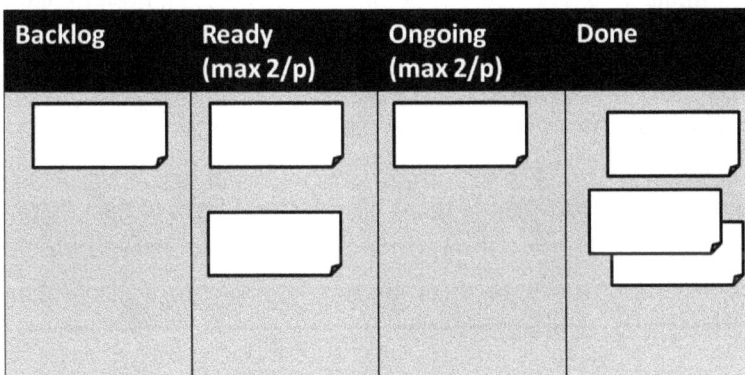

Whenever you create a new task, you write it down on a sticky note and put it in the Backlog column. There can be any number of tasks waiting in the Backlog. Then you select a number of tasks to put in the Ready column. These are tasks that you, or someone else, is about to start. Put a limit on this column; stick to 2 or 3 tasks per person. When you start working on a task, write your name on the sticky note and put it in the Ongoing column. Again, **there may be only 1 or 2 tasks in Ongoing per person.** Finally, when a task is done, you move it to the Done column, where it stays as long as needed.

What's important about this is that you limit the number of tasks in the Ready and Ongoing columns to numbers that you can handle.

Check the Kanban board at least once per day

This board business is all very cool, but quite useless if you don't also use it to get things done. It helps to put it in a location where you can see it as often as possible — but don't let it blend into the environment. Put it in your office, in plain view. Put it in your kitchen. Put it anywhere — just not in the bathroom.

Urgent work

A possibility is to have two Kanban boards, or one split up horizontally in two sections: one for Urgent tasks and one for Normal tasks. For Urgent tasks, the limit would be 1 task per column per person. Of course you also need to decide what the criteria are for defining a task as urgent. I'll leave that up to you, as it depends on so many factors. As long as the tasks that end up on that board are very urgent, and do not take the focus off the other tasks unnecessarily. It is perfectly fine not to have any urgent tasks on the board for quite a while, so resist the urge to promote every task to an Urgent one, even if the Urgent board is empty.

Color-coding again

It's a good idea to use sticky notes of different colors; say, standard yellow for standard tasks and blue or pink for urgent ones. You will automatically gravitate towards the urgent tasks, and you can tell if there's any urgent work just by glimpsing at the Kanban board.

Not for planning

Notice that Kanban is not a planning tool; it is a tracking tool. There is no particular order in which to perform the tasks, and there is no deadline per task. Rather, it gives an overview of what is done, what is ongoing and what is to come.

Keep Track of Important Documents

At home, you can use a filing cabinet to keep copies of important documents (see also "Part 2 : Dealing with Clutter"). But in order to keep track of *all* important documents – whether they are personal or business – and to have them "at your fingertips" always, you can also use an electronic system. And best of all, it's (nearly) free.

Electronic

To begin with, use as many electronic documents as possible. I prefer to receive invoices as PDF files via e-mail; that is a first archive of documents right there.

If you do get the documents on paper, scan them so that they become PDF or TIFF files. You'll have to invest in a scanner/copier/printer, but nowadays these are really cheap.

E-mail archive

Next, send all of your important documents, once they are in electronic form, to a special online e-mail-address. For example, if you like to use the Windows Live Mail service, you may create an address such as *john.doe.archive@live.com*.

Use tags (short search terms) in the body of the mail message. For instance, if you have received a hotel invoice, send it to your archive address with

Hotel Invoice: Caribbean Inn (summer 2011)

as the subject line, and in the body, write tags such as

hotel bill, vacation, Kingston, Jamaica, 2011-08-01, August, $930

Now when you need to retrieve a particular invoice, or this one, later, just log on to your online archive e-mail account and search for one or more of these search terms and *voilà!* The invoice is there; you can view it online or download it to your PC and print it.

It's important that you enter any tags you can think of which might be useful when searching.

The beauty of this solution is that your documents are now available everywhere; not just at home or at the office, but *everywhere* – even if you're on the train in the middle of nowhere and need to know *pronto* how much you paid for electricity last year (assuming, of course, that you carry an Internet-enabled device).

When sending very important mails

When you send a very important mail, especially one that includes an important document, quietly *bcc* (blind carbon copy) it to your archive account as well. You'll then always know where to find it.

"Back up" your important cards too

"Important documents" also means your credit cards, membership cards and the like. Scan them all on both sides and send the scans to your archive e-mail address. You never know when you might need them, and if you lose your cards at least you can identify them.

PART 2

DEALING WITH CLUTTER

Reduce Clutter by Letting Go

Letting go of stuff is hard, especially for us. It seems we always want to hold on to things. We keep the stuff we know we should get rid of because we assume it may come in handy later, or we have an emotional connection to it. But what is the result? We clutter up our environments. We dump stuff we never use or even look at in boxes, closets, and the car. I'm not just talking about old receipts or childhood toys.

Look around you and see what clutters up your bedroom, your living room, your car, your garage, your office:

- Old magazines and newspapers
- Travel souvenirs
- Gifts (wanted or unwanted)
- Photo frames
- Pictures and photo books from previous relationships
- Old clothes that no longer fit
- Old shoes
- Old toys the kids have outgrown
- Old briefcases (one from the era of 15" laptops, another for 17" laptops, another...)
- Old cell phones, cameras, and other devices you paid good money for but no longer use (or worse, that no longer *work!*)
- Refrigerator magnets that hold out-of-date coupons, drawings your youngest made a year ago and letters that "remind" you to pay bills
- Heaps and heaps of old plastic bags and cardboard boxes
- ...

Just imagine that – poof! – all that stuff disappeared. No more piles and boxes in the hallway that you have to maneuver around just to get to the bathroom. No more stacks of old paperwork and "magazines to read" that you know you'll never get to anyway. Only the stuff you use and need. You'll have a clear kitchen table, a floor you can see, a garage that you can actually use to park your car.

Doesn't that sound good? Doesn't this prospect make you feel better already?

Even though it seems all of this stuff adds value to your life, most of it doesn't. A cluttered environment is a source of worry, stress and frustration, and so the best thing to do about it is to **get rid of everything that doesn't add value.** Anything that isn't essential and that doesn't really tug at your heart should go. What remains is easier to organize, and you'll have less stuff to worry about.

What is essential?

If you've kept something in a box in your garage for a year, how essential is it? And if you hold on to last week's newspaper because it may contain interesting articles or useable coupons, then either you should read those articles and cut those coupons, or just throw away the paper. It's no use holding on to things because they may come in handy later. We all do this, but it's a waste of time and space. Get rid of that clutter.

So, room by room, corner by corner, set some time aside regularly to clean up and get rid of what is not essential. You may instead decide to sweep through the house in one go ("clean-up weekend"), and if that works for you, fine. For me, it's a lot easier to do it in small manageable increments. I regularly do some clean-up and decluttering work for, say, 20 to 30 minutes. That keeps it attainable.

Either way, it pays to get help when getting rid of all the cluttering stuff. Do it together with your partner, a friend or a parent, or whomever you know is well-organized and honest enough to tell you to throw something away when you have to (see also "Build a Support System").

When "doing" a room, decide what is essential and what you can give away to a friend or a charity (or sell in a garage sale). Everything else is garbage. Essential things stay. Garbage goes, no excuses. The rest you can set aside for a short time to give away or sell. Give yourself no more than a week or so to get rid of it, or it becomes clutter again!

Give Everything its Own Place

When life hands you chaos, make chaosade.

I'm not even sure that's a word, but basically what this means is that we are inherently chaotic and therefore must reduce the chaos, including clutter, out of our lives as much as possible. Clutter in the house does cause clutter in the mind, and frustration, and problems finding important things back such as bills, pens, and keys.

The #2 technique to reduce clutter (after "Letting go") is to give everything its own place: one place, where it logically belongs, so you know where to look for it.

For example: where are your *keys* right now? Mine are in the right-front pocket of my pants. No matter where I am, no matter day or night, no matter the month or the year: my keys are always in the same spot. I never have to look for them. I only take them out to use them (or when I switch clothes) and as soon as I can, I put them back where they belong.

My cell phone? In the left-front pocket of my pants.

The remote? On the Mickey Mouse table next to the TV.

Pens? In the pen holder on the desktop.

Scissors? In the top-left kitchen drawer, front section. (I actually have scissors on every floor of the house – that's another trick – but that is where the scissors are on the first floor).

And so on, and so on.

What you need to do is pick a logical spot, practical and easy to remember, and then stick to that choice. This means that, when you've used an item, you put it back where it belongs as soon as possible. Otherwise, it's no use giving it its own place.

Your pockets

Your pockets are an excellent place to keep things you need all the time. I already mentioned that I have fixed pockets for my cell phone, my keys and my wallet. I have another easy to remember place: my key ring. It is in fact a tiny Leatherman Micra multi-tool. I carry this handy gizmo with me all the time and I never have to look for small scissors, a file, a straight screwdriver, a bottle opener etc. It's super-handy.

What is especially interesting about having an implement such as this with you all the time is that it takes away excuses for procrastination. Yes, you *can* open that box *right now:* you have scissors and a small knife on you. Yes, you *can* unscrew those screws and replace that battery, *right now*... And so on.

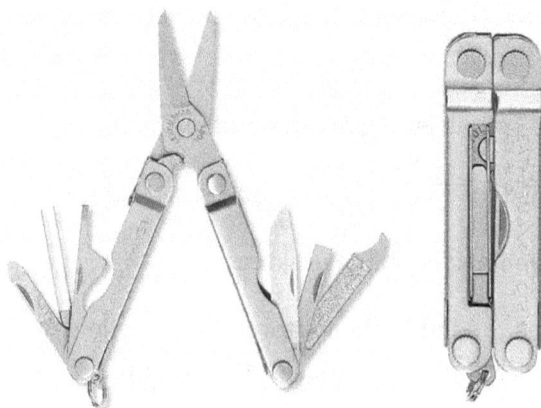

Your handbag

Whereas gents usually have pockets, ladies tend to have handbags. In your handbag, too, everything should have its own place. It's no use turning your handbag into a carry-on Dumpster. Limit what you carry and know where to put it. You'll never have to dig for lipstick or your cell phone again.

All tied up

Chris is a very busy businessman, and he runs a print shop. He and his coworkers constantly work with all kinds of tools and implements. One day he got so tired of always having to look for cutters and scissors that he tied them to the desks with string. Each string is long enough to allow comfortable use, but the tools can never get lost.

In every room or on every floor

Another way to make sure you don't have to run far to get the things you need is to have them everywhere. In my house, there are designated places for scissors and pens on every floor. In the same fashion, give teens their own tools and make them responsible for them – so that they won't run off with your stuff.

Keep a list

You may want to write up a list of where everything goes in case you tend to forget. Very soon, you'll start reaping the benefits.

Reduce Visual Clutter

Visual clutter, unsurprisingly, is visible chaos. It's that bookshelf with the mix of standing and lying, big and small books. It's the empty can on your desk, the toys on the floor, the disorganized stack of papers on top of the filing cabinet.

Visual clutter is not clutter per se – you may need those documents, and you do need to sort through them. You need those books even though you can probably give some of them away. But when you look around, you see disharmony and chaos. Your brain must work harder to process the images, and you'll feel less at peace. Visual clutter is just as disturbing as actual clutter. So get rid of it.

Closets with doors and boxes with lids

Hide the visual clutter behind doors, lids and curtains. When you buy a new cabinet, pick one with doors or with plastic boxes that fill up the open spaces.

Keep a "treasure chest" with a lid close by. Then when you get visitors, quickly dump all visual clutter in the chest. This is also a good solution when you have small children; if they cannot yet clean up their toys properly, you can have them put their toys in the chest before they go to bed.

The net result will be a quieter environment and more peace of mind.

Don't Turn Your Living Room or Bedroom into Something Else

We're still on the subject of clutter, but looking at it from a different angle. Do you have a desk with a computer, filing cabinets and piles of paperwork in your living room or your bedroom? If so, you're turning that space into an office. This attracts clutter where it doesn't belong, and reduces the quality of the time you spend in those rooms.

We have trouble with duality

There are of course many good reasons to do this. Using part of the living room as office space means you can spend more time with the kids or your partner while you're working. The same is true for the computer in the bedroom. But this is precisely the kind of duality that we have a hard time dealing with. We don't want piles of paperwork in the living room, do we? We certainly don't want our kids to practice their coloring or origami skills on our bills. And we definitely want a clear separation between work time and free time.

Havens

Similarly, when having a desk with a computer in the bedroom, that bedroom is no longer a haven of peace and quiet. It becomes a workplace. It becomes hard – if not impossible – to let go of work, slow down your brain and get to sleep in that workplace.

Consequently, if you can, put that desk in a dedicated room. Living rooms are living rooms and bedrooms are bedrooms, nothing else.

One box of toys in the living room

If you have small kids, you'll be familiar with the image of boxes and toys spread all over the living room as if a tornado just ran through it. But the living room is not a den. Training the kids to pick up after themselves is one possible tactic; another is to try to get them to put away the toys they just finished playing with before they play with other toys (see also "Reduce Visual Clutter").

But a golden rule is to have one, and only one, box of toys in the living room. If the children want to play with other toys in the living room, they can, but first they'll have to make room in that box. This keeps the total potential tornado debris to a known minimum. Granted, this works best with kids who are old enough to take on some responsibility.

Newspapers and magazines

Throw away books, magazines and newspapers you know you'll never read (again). Alternatively, you can use two boxes: **Almost Going** and **Going**. Put every book, newspaper or magazine you're not sure you want to throw away yet in the *Almost Going* box.

Every two weeks, you empty the *Going* box in the trash, and you move everything from the *Almost Going* box to *Going*. That gives you up to a month to take action and read. After that, it's clear that the book or magazine is just clutter, and out it goes.

Replace books by their e-book versions

I used to have two bookcases full of books. Rows and rows of books, most of which I had either already read and would never read again (but I kept them just in case), and others which I planned to read but never got around to.

One day, after wanting a proper e-reader for some time, I decided to take the plunge. I ordered a Kindle, Amazon's e-reader, and I haven't looked back since. This was one of the best decisions I ever made.

I gave away the books I knew I'd never read anyway, and those I knew I'd read if I had the time – on the condition that there was an e-book version of the book available. Luckily, the library of available e-books is growing rapidly, so most books I was planning to read were available already.

Now I always have at least one Kindle with me. There are at least sixty books on it, and downloading a new title takes only 60 seconds. When talking about instant gratification, the Kindle is it. But more importantly, I can read any book I want at any time without having to carry two bookcases on my back, and there's never any clutter with half-read books lying around everywhere. Since switching to an e-reader, I get a lot more reading done. Really, this was one of the best decisions I ever made.

Filing Cabinets to the Rescue

To properly organize all the clutter in your home or office, you need filing cabinets. You can get these in a variety of forms, sizes and prices at many vendors such as Ikea.

A good filing cabinet comes with drawers. Really, a shelf or rack is better than nothing but it's still visual clutter. If you can put everything away neatly into drawers, that is so much nicer. To find the correct drawer swiftly, use a label maker (see also "The Label Maker is Your Friend").

I find it useful if the drawers or transparent or, better, semi-transparent. Even if they are labeled (and mine all are), it's still convenient that you can actually see what's in there, without it becoming visual clutter.

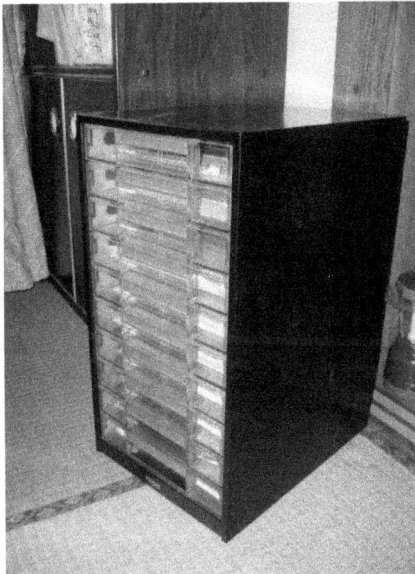

At work

At work, I keep a mini filing cabinet on my desk with separate drawers for medications, change, cables (I am an IT consultant, what can I say?) and stationary.

At home

Some filing cabinets you can even stack. I have 12 of such stackable, all-plastic, transparent-drawer filing cabinets at home, each with five drawers.

I have drawers for virtually everything you can think of. Here is a random selection:

- Audio/Video Cables
- Documents related to the house: Blueprints, bank documents and notary documents
- Electric cables
- Lamps: Contains regular bulbs as well as stick-on LED lights
- Mail: Contains envelopes, birthday cards, condolence cards, and stamps
- PC Cables: Contains mostly USB cables in many forms and sizes
- PC-Related Hardware: Contains webcam and small sound amplifiers currently not in use. (Come to think of it, I may have to let go of these...)
- Phone: Contains the manual, a cable to connect the phone to the PC, and a box with my previous phone
- Photo Camera: Includes the camera itself, cables, spare batteries, and manual
- Power strips
- Printer: Contains printing paper, a few ink cartridges and a DVD with driver software for my printer
- Software (Microsoft): Contains DVDs and manuals
- Software (non-Microsoft): Contains DVDs and manuals

- Video Camera: Contains the video camera (and my previous one), cables, and manual
- Warranty Cards

Desk filing cabinets

Desk filing cabinets are handy *for In/Out drawers* and generally for the documents you work with daily, and for stationary (pens, pencils, sticky notes, and the like).

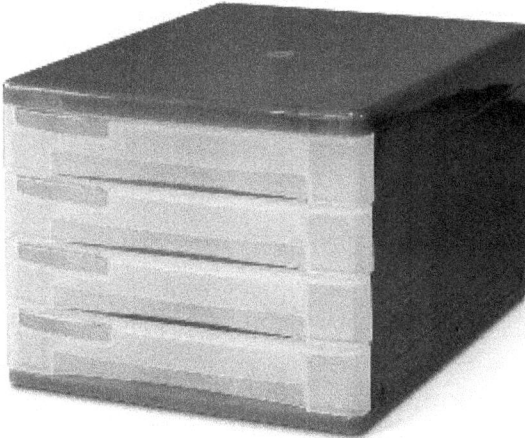

The toolbox

You can get a toolbox that comes with lots of little boxes and containers. If you need to look for a particular size of nail or screw, put them in their own separate containers and *label* them clearly.

Lost and Found

You can use a drawer, or a box with a lid on, as a **Lost & Found** box. Whenever you find something in the house where it doesn't belong, and you don't know where it belongs (it happens), put it in there. The person who lost the item will, after countless hours of fruitless searching (or a quick enquiry) look for it there.

Electronics for Clutter Management

Here are a few examples of electronic aids to clutter management:

House-cleaning robots

If you're into nifty electronics, you probably already have one of those super-handy house-cleaning robots. I have one to vacuum and another to wash the floor with detergent. You can get robots like these (mine are built by IRobot; see also *http://www.irobot.com*) at most electronics stores.

House-cleaning robots don't always do a perfect job and they don't replace your housework, but they do reduce it significantly. Turn on the vacuuming robot right before you leave the house—they are as noisy as regular vacuum cleaners. But you'll have more time to waste on fun things. I also guarantee fewer arguments over chores when these handy helpers are around.

Washer/Dryer Combos

If you keep forgetting to take the laundry out of the washer and put it in the dryer, then the Washer/Dryer Combo is for you. These machines, which cost about as much as a washing machine plus a drying machine, take up less space and do both jobs in a single go. Just select the wash cycle and the dry cycle and you're good to go. Remember when it's time to get those clothes out, or they'll wrinkle anyway.

PART 3

MONEY MATTERS

Budgeting to Track and Keep Your Money

It is common knowledge that money is easier to manage by using a specialized computerized system such as **Quicken** or **Microsoft Money**. These computer programs help you to keep track of expenses and to budget per category; for instance, you may plan to set aside $100 per month for medical expenses, $90 for entertainment, etc. You make up the categories as you see fit. You keep track of your expenses per category, so that you can adjust when necessary and keep from spending more than you make. That sounds straightforward and I'm sure that to many people, it's a lifesaver. For our gang, it may or may not be enough.

The Dedicated Accounts System

ADDer Bea taught me her way to set and keep money aside per category. I modified it slightly and call it the *Dedicated Accounts System.* The idea is very simple: you create a set of checking and/or savings accounts, one per expense category. Many banks offer free checking, and moving money into and out of a checking account is relatively easy, so this is what I use.

Now, in our family we have worked out approximately how much we must or can spend per category per month. For instance, we put away a certain amount per month in a joint savings account, we put aside 1/12 of our estimated yearly recurring costs, we stash $100 per month for entertainment, etc. The idea is that we create a separate checking account per category. In the beginning of the month, we transfer the money in the "general" joint checking account to all those different accounts. When we go to the movie theater, we pay for the tickets with the Entertainment account. We pay the energy bills with the Energy and Water Account, and toys we buy with money from... You know what I mean.

Adjusting

When account is empty, it's empty. For some categories that's okay – if there's no more money for online poker, you just have to wait it out until next month. But if there's no more money to pay for necessities, you'll have to transfer money from the other accounts to the correct account, and adjust the spread of money next month. That's why it is a good idea to start out conservatively and to assign more money than you think is necessary to necessities and less money to categories that are less needed. Don't gamble with the rent, you know the principle.

Autopay

Use autopay to pay your recurring bills such as electricity, gas, Internet, and the like. The beauty of this is that it is so simple to do and you never get fined for not paying on time. This is another example of using automation to simplify things and get the boring work over with.

Magic Markers

Before you file a bill or invoice, mark both the date and the amount to pay with a magic marker. When you have to sift through a whole stack of invoices later, you'll be happy to quickly find this information.

Impulse Control when Shopping – or, "Do I *Really* Want This?"

One day, I went into a music store for some information, and walked out with a $2,000 guitar. Sound familiar? Read on.

Buy me!

So, I went into the music store, because I was interested in learning how to achieve a particular sound on the guitar. I was thinking of components, special-effect boxes, or just proper technique. The salesman told me that to get the authentic sound I was looking for, I needed a particular type of guitar. He showed me and I was so enchanted that I bought it on the spot. Later that night, I couldn't sleep because I realized that I had been too impulsive, even though my new purchase sounded exactly like what I was looking for.

I should have remembered the lesson I got from my friend Sandra. When I was in college, Sandra, a fellow student, taught me how she bought clothes. She would try them on, take a quick look in the mirror, and listen if the clothes would beg: *"Buy me, buy me, buy me!"* If so, she would buy them; otherwise, she would return the clothes to the rack and move on.

She was right, of course. I took her advice to heart, and this simple habit has served me well in the past years. It has saved me thousands of dollars, and I have started using for other goods as well. Why is it so effective? Because it lowers the chance of *impulse buying*.

I hear you counter – *"What if* everything *I try on begs purchase?"* Then you're not listening hard enough to the voice. You're just kidding yourself. The *"buy me, buy me, buy me"* voice must come immediately when you glance in the mirror, otherwise it's just an afterthought.

Want it three times

This is another method I use, mostly for expensive things that catch my eye. Shiny, slick, just-out stuff promises to make me happy, if only for a few days. A TV with a screen 2 inches wider than mine? A new media player with twice the memory of the one I have? A new camcorder, a comfy lounger with massage function or a new computer? I find all of those hard to resist.

The technique is this: I want something, I recognize that fact, and I also recognize that I'm probably being impulsive. I decide *not to buy it* if I don't absolutely *need it* right away. Then, if I find myself wanting to buy the same item again later – say, at least one week later – then again I wonder if I can live without it for another while. Usually I have to admit that, yes, life will be bearable without the purchase. And, finally, if I find myself wanting to buy the same item a *third* time, again with enough time in-between, I go ahead and buy it. I should have used this technique when faced with the guitar.

How do you understand that you don't absolutely need this item? Well, ask yourself this: "How did I find this item – was it something I was actively looking for, or was it something I bumped into?" If it's the latter, you can live without it, at least for a while.

Get objective information

Buying on impulse tends to mean "responding to ads and infomercials." Yet, these can hardly be mistaken for objective sources of information. So, common sense tells us to avoid ads and especially infomercials, which are just long commercials disguised as objective information. I *never* watch infomercials, they make me cringe.

But there is a lot of objective information within reach. If you're looking to buy something specific, go online and find as many reviews as you can. No matter what type of purchase you are contemplating, do your research. If you want to find out about a certain model of a certain device, Google that model name and you'll find a lot of information. Focus on data coming from consumer organizations and user forums. The consumer organizations are very objective and look at the products they review from many angles. In user forums you can learn from those who have already made the purchase.

To find reviews for almost any product, I like to consult Amazon.com. They allow everyone to post reviews, positive or negative. Another interesting site is ConsumerSearch.com. For books, you can also find many reviews at Barnes & Noble (BN.com).

Read at least two positive and two negative reviews before you decide whether to purchase the item.

Pay cash

It may be that not spending money is difficult for you. If that's the case, make sure that when you're out, you can't kill yourself financially. Bring only a limited amount of money, and pay cash as often as possible. The reason for this is that you actually see how much you're spending. A credit card is invisible money, and invisible money flies away faster and easier than tangible cash. See also "The Low-Limit Credit Card."

The Low-Limit Credit Card

Kim is a prime example of an ADD sufferer who has issues with not spending money. That is, once armed with a credit card, she can do serious damage without even realizing it. That is why she decided, after some counseling, to lower her credit card limit. This automatically took care of most of the issue: sure she can have a spending spree, but then it's all over until next month. This quickly resulted in being more money-aware and, of course, it keeps the monthly bill to a known max.

Credit cards are black holes of debt

Realize that **credit-card expenditures are in fact debts.** You're spending invisible money, but the bill will come and it will put a dent in your budget. Every cent you spend on something you don't need, is money thrown away. On top of your spending, the credit card companies charge a hefty interest for the privilege of using their plastic. All of this builds up and if you thus outspend your income, it's going to result in huge problems for a long time to come. If this is an issue you are facing, get rid of all of your credit cards but the lowest-limit one today.

Statements

To keep spending from running out of control, it also helps to actually **read your monthly statements.** This way you may discover recurring debits that you thought were canceled, such as automatically-extended memberships. You may also discover credit card fraud early enough to stop it from ruining you.

And, again, if you have trouble with this, let a trusted friend or accountant help you.

Some More Money Tips

Spare change

I like to keep spare change in the house and the car for emergencies. Regularly, I "dump" some change from my pockets in a small container in the house, or the one in my car, so that I always have some money with me. It never builds up to more than $50, but that is enough to cover most small unexpected expenses, such as parking meters, quick bites, or gas.

The organized wallet

I am a freelancer, and so I carry around a personal credit card as well as a business credit card. Likewise, I have a whole set of membership and other cards that are either personal or business. So I have organized my wallet hence.

When I fold open my wallet, my personal cards are on the left and my business cards are on the right. This makes it easy for me to keep things separate and to find back the right card quickly.

Pay invoices electronically as much as you can

This is fast and convenient, especially if you receive them in your e-mailbox. You can also immediately print out a proof of payment when necessary.

Make a habit of paying invoices as soon as you get them

If that is difficult financially, check the expiration date of the invoice and schedule the payment at least a week before that. Really pay them when that date arrives; you don't want to waste good money on late fees and interests, and you don't want to be known as the person who seldom pays on time.

Paying immediately buys you goodwill. You may get an immediate reduction, or at some later time, your creditors may remember how timely you've always paid and cut you some slack when you need it.

PART 4

DEALING WITH PROCRASTINATION

I'll Do it Tomorrow

Man, if I had a million dollars for every time I've said that... Even for many non-ADD people, procrastination is a way of life. It is a way of not having to deal with tasks that are cumbersome, boring or potentially sobering – such as doing our taxes, opening a bill, or even just opening the mailbox.

The dictionary defines **pro·cras·ti·na·tion** as

To put off doing something, especially out of habitual carelessness or laziness.

We tend to replace one timely task by another, less timely task. It seems there are many reasons to procrastinate, but the most common may be that we want to avoid something boring, or daunting. I remember that, as a college student, I found all kinds of important things to do when I knew I should have been studying topics that didn't really interest me.

We like to act as if, by not doing anything, the task we don't want to face will go away all by itself and we'll be fine. But if we find the task unpleasant, why would it get any better by delaying? It won't. The longer we wait, the worse it gets. Procrastination is something we have to get rid of, ADD or not.

Using peer pressure to your advantage

One technique to counter procrastination is by doing the work with a partner. If you tend to bail out of administration work, book some time with an accountant or someone else who might help you. This makes the work less unpleasant and the peer pressure you create makes it much harder to escape. And what are you going to do when a friend comes over to help you shape up your garden?

We need deadlines

Another technique to counter procrastination is the use of a deadline. Did you ever notice that, when you had a deadline, at the last moment you suddenly did get the rush to do what you had to do? Of course there's still the element of the last minute, but at least the task got done.

Deadlines should be clear. A good deadline must:

- define the task to do;
- define the exact date and time the task must be completed;
- be realistic: don't tell yourself to paint all rooms in the house in one day. Unrealistic deadlines lead to predictable failure and, hence, more procrastination.

Write down the deadline, put it in your calendar and make sure your smartphone reminds you of the task at hand.

Self-imposed deadlines

So if you don't have a deadline in order to complete a task, one thing you can do is impose one yourself. Tell yourself to perform a particular task before bedtime, or before Thursday noon.

True, a self-imposed deadline is not as powerful as one imposed by someone else or by circumstances. But there are some techniques you can use to enhance their power.

Penalties and Rewards

Deadlines don't work if there's no penalty for missing the deadline. Likewise, they work better if there is a reward for making the deadline. So if you want to impose deadlines on yourself, make sure there is a penalty and a reward.

A good penalty

A good example of a penalty for missing a deadline is that you must do another task on your to-do list immediately (how's that for a motivator?) A penalty must be unpleasant, but not too much so and it should not penalize anyone but you. Accordingly, not taking the kids out to the playground is not a good penalty for you. The penalty/effort for making the deadline must also make sense, of course; it's no use giving yourself 25 lashes for not washing the car before Monday.

A good reward

Likewise, the reward/effort ratio must be sensible. You're not going to reward yourself with a trip to Disney World for filing your taxes on time. But you may reward yourself that way for filing all of your paperwork, including tax returns, in time for 3 years in a row.

Rewards can be financial (allow yourself some extra spending money), or about family (spend more time with your kids, spend a romantic weekend together in a spa, go to an amusement park), very simple (a double dose of sweetener in your coffee), or anything you can think of.

But don't take it all too seriously

The penalty-and-reward system's purpose is to help you lower your tendency to procrastinate, and hence to get things actually done. But don't tie your self-worth to it. When it all becomes too difficult, cut yourself some slack and switch to another strategy – such as enlisting others to help you. See also "Build a Support System" in this book.

Don't Be Late, Now

How often have you heard that one? People who know you already expect you to be late. Here are a few tactics to counter those expectations:

Set your calendar early – but not always

In "10 Reasons to invest in a smartphone", another chapter of this book, I explain how I use Google Calendar on the Web and on my phone. I enter appointments or events as soon as I know about them, and I invite others to the appointment as necessary.

One of the things I also do, then, is to set the start time a bit early. I may have an appointment at 8 PM, but I'll put in 7:45 or even 7:30 in my calendar. This simple trick helps to get there on time.

What makes this tactic even better is that I don't *always* use it. Sometimes an 8 PM appointment really means an 8 PM appointment. But I put so many things in my calendar – including taking the garbage out – that I cannot remember which start times are accurate and which are not. So, I do my best to be on time, and often I have some buffer time that I wasn't even aware of.

Estimate time more conservatively and add 10%

I find that it does help to estimate the time needed to get there more conservatively. I expect traffic problems, parking problems and the necessary delay when traveling with young children.

Try to estimate the time accurately, add 10%, and take that time as the reminder period for your appointments. For instance, say that you have a doctor's appointment at 7 PM. You estimate that, from home, you need 20 minutes to get to the doctor (including time to park and walk), and 5 minutes to get ready. So that is a 25-minute lead, plus 10% = 27 ½ minutes. Therefore, let your calendar remind you about the appointment 30 minutes before start time, and you'll probably be fine. You can even choose to add another safety buffer and get reminded some 40 minutes before the appointment. But beware – buffer time is no reason to slack.

Let me just quickly...

Ouch. How often are we ADDers late because, right before we had to leave, we said: "let me just quickly finish this, and then I'll be on my way..."? Only to leave at least 20 minutes late, with the known results. This temptation is hard to resist, but realize this:

- Any task that you think you'll finish quickly, takes longer than you think – if not *double* the amount of time that you planned.
- ADDers are notoriously bad at estimating required time to finish a task. It's as if we are incorrigible optimists, time-wise.

So when you catch yourself saying, "let me just quickly finish this...", then double your time estimate and see if this is really what you want to do.

Calling when you're late

It is a good habit to call when you're running late. As soon as you realize you'll be late for an appointment, call to let the other person(s) know how late you expect to arrive. It's better to estimate a later arrival than an earlier one, as it is more likely that you'll hit a later target.

If you're running late when returning home, it's also a good idea to call those who are waiting for you – such as your partner, parents, or friends. But our brains are often so busy (especially when we're focused on work) that we forget to let our loved ones at home know that we'll be later. Therefore, it is a better habit to *always* call when you leave for home. This, again, adds structure to your day and improves communication with the home front. When you're running late, they will know about it, and there will be less frustration.

The "Do It Now" Attitude

When looking for excuses to procrastinate, try this: tell yourself to "do it now". Realize, there and then, that you're just looking for reasons to postpone and that there is no time like the present. Then get up and do it. This is what William Knaus, in his excellent book **End Procrastination Now**, calls the **"Do It Now" Attitude**.

It takes some work to make this second nature, and surely you'll often have to remind yourself, but saying "do it now" and then *making it happen,* makes you feel really good afterward. The satisfaction of actually having beaten the habit is immense, and you'll have much less damage control to deal with later. You'll also have less stress, because real stress comes from the weight of your **In** box.

Do it now. Now is best.

Don't get discouraged

Of course it is difficult to adopt a new mindset. It will take time, and that is OK. The key is to catch yourself *dismissing* the idea to "do it now" in time. Don't let yourself get away with it.

Understand that once you *start* doing what you want to procrastinate, the hard part is over. Once you are doing it, you have conquered your own resistance.

But if you fail to catch yourself dismissing that idea, don't get discouraged. Do not think that the mindset is not for you and that you will always be a procrastinator. Instead, promise yourself to work on it, and really try your best. Apply the reward system and if you have to, the penalty system too. Ask someone to remind you what you need to do. Ask to really get on your case if necessary.

Whatever you do, do not give up. You will pick up the habit.

Electronics for Time Management

Here are some convenient electronic time management helpers:

Kitchen timer

Kitchen timers are not only useful in the kitchen. If my friend Bea only has ten minutes to take a shower, she sets a kitchen timer to 9 minutes right before she hops in, and she won't lose track of time dreaming away under the soothing water. Now get that image out of your head, back to kitchen timers.

These little inexpensive gizmos can also help you get started on a task you dislike. It takes some discipline (or better yet, an accomplice) to set the time and to actually do it once the timer rings, but I find it does help. "When the timer goes off, I'll start on the dishes." Of course I mean I'll put the plates in the dishwasher, but you know what I'm trying to say.

If you're the parent of an ADD kid, rejoice that kitchen timers work wonders with ADD kids who need to stop doing something they like. Give them ample warning, say, 10 minutes: "Robin, you can play on your Xbox until the timer rings, and then we're having dinner…"

Smartphone

If you're technically inclined, a smartphone can be a big help to organize your life.

Smartphones typically carry Calendar software that is compatible with popular PC formats such as Microsoft Outlook. This means that, if you connect your phone to your PC at least daily, your calendar will stay in sync between your PC(s) and your phone. This way, you can be reminded all day long about upcoming appointments, meetings, etc., and you can look up what's coming. You can also write down any upcoming appointments and reminders, and they will be uploaded to your computer the next time you connect, or to the Internet immediately.

With the on-board Internet browser, you can read mail, consult the train or bus schedule, etc. Phones with GPS are extra handy, because you'll never get lost and you can usually look up the nearest gas station, restaurants, and so forth.

The bad thing about using a smartphone is that you can get so hooked on it, that it starts to control you rather than the other way around. If you have or will get a smartphone, keep in mind that it's only a device to help you organize your life – your life does not revolve around it.

Radio-controlled watch

A radio-controlled watch is always right. No matter daylight saving time, no matter if it's a leap year, it always tells the time and date right all by itself.

It's also handy to have radio-controlled wall clocks and alarm clocks. It saves those precious minutes when daylight saving time changes and at least you'll have clocks that all agree on the time.

PART 5

REDUCING STRESS

Perfection Doesn't Exist – Accept "Good Enough"

One of the mixed blessings of ADD is perfectionism. This trait enables us to really shine and rise beyond all expectations. It drives us to do our jobs with the utmost meticulous attention to detail. Never mind food and sleep when we're hyper-focused, the result will be worth it.

Except that this perfectionism of ours is really a curse. Perfectionism is not healthy and tends to be bad for relationships. Dr. Prem Fry, a psychology professor at Trinity Western University in Canada, studied this phenomenon and commented, "Perfectionism is a virtue to be extolled definitely. But beyond a certain threshold, it backfires and becomes an impediment."

One problem is that our perfectionism doesn't end when we leave work and go home. We set a high bar not only for ourselves, but also for our loved ones and everyone else. It wears us out and puts a strain on our relationships.

Self-worth

Another problem is that we are often not happy with work we deliver, even though it is good enough. We doubt ourselves, we toss and turn over details that nobody even notices. We tie our self-worth to our performance. We think we are failures if we don't produce perfect results. This causes us not only to procrastinate more, but we also get a completely distorted view of what's important. We may even lose control when under stress. The net effect is that because of our perfectionism, we get less done!

In *10 Simple Solutions to Adult ADD,* Dr. Stephanie Sarkis writes, "Remember, even people without ADD are not perfect. Give yourself a break, and allow yourself to relax. Set challenging yet achievable goals for yourself".

It's physically unhealthy

In an extensive study, the aforementioned Dr. Fry looked at the relationship between perfectionism and physical health. She found that people who placed high expectations on themselves to be perfect, had a 51% increased risk of early death over people who did not.

In short: perfectionists die younger.

The study also showed some positive results of perfectionism: diabetes type 2 patients who were perfectionists generally lived longer than those who were not perfectionists – probably due to their taking better care of themselves.

Accept "good enough"

So, when is good enough good enough? Ask others for input. Take the writing of this book as an example. If I wanted it to be perfect, you would still not be reading it. Instead, I wrote and wrote, rewrote, modified, deleted and wrote again. In the meantime I asked a number of ADD colleagues to review the drafts. When they said it was good, I accepted that rather than re-polishing or starting all over again.

Accepting "good enough" lowers stress levels. It even improves our self-esteem because we get more done.

Remember this:

Work is good enough when, in the perception of the target group, it is good.

One Thing at a Time; You're Not a Juggler

One of the things we with our racecar minds are all guilty of is having too many simultaneous projects. Whenever we get a really great idea (and that happens all of the time, bless our souls), we cannot wait to get started and put everything else on hold. Soon we leave a trail of abandoned projects, semi-active projects and the one really cool *Project of the Moment.*

You know what's coming next. Our minds are not just racecars; they're also mostly one-track (especially for us menfolk). One-track minds should stick to single simultaneous projects, maybe two if time allows. But what we need help with is to keep our focus on that one project, even though we are already thinking of the next cool thing which is infinitely more interesting than what we are doing now.

For this, keep the following in mind: **Whatever we are doing or working on right now, it seemed a really great idea "at the time".** So what happened? Why are we not giving that great idea all we have? How often are we going to put it on hold? Are we ever going to finish it? If we're never going to finish it, it was all just a waste of time and we're never going to see our vision – any vision – come to life.

Force yourself to focus on one project. Enlist the help of others; maybe to help finish the project, or just to keep you on track.

- Do you have an idea for a book, and you really think you can pull it off? Get the word out to proofreaders, and get some work out the door as soon as you can. Have them ponder on you for fresh and regular updates. Use that pressure to make sure you keep writing.

- Do you still need to paint the bedroom? Put it in your calendar, make sure you keep the time available, and have someone come over to help you. Surely you can ask your significant other, but there's more pressure on you to actually do it if someone else is involved who puts his or her precious time aside to help you out.

You can use a Kanban board to measure your progress and to keep your focus on the one or two projects. See also "Kanban: To-Do Lists on Steroids" in this book.

One thing at a time, any time

This tactic also works on another dimension: immediate time. It's very hard, if not impossible, to handle two things at once. We humans need to focus in order to do something properly, and we cannot focus on two things at once. That is why we cannot answer phone calls and drive at the same time (at least not without significant danger to ourselves and the other drivers). Scientists have discovered that when people focus on a single task, both halves of the *medial frontal cortex* of the brain work together. But when people try to handle two simultaneous tasks, each half focuses on one of those, and consequently the quality of the work diminishes. Three simultaneous tasks becomes a more serious problem as it is mathematically proven that the medial frontal cortex consists of only two halves.

This phenomenon also seems to be at the root of the fact that humans have difficulty choosing between more than two options. (The study was conducted by Prof. Sylvain Charron and Prof. Etienne Koechlin, both of France's National Institute of Health and Medical Research.)

Handling interruptions

Often, of course, you get interrupted. You were doing something, or were on your way to do something, and then something else pops up that requires your immediate attention. Such interruptions can be frustrating, especially for us ADDers, who have problems context switching *and then switching back*. That is the hardest part – returning to what you were doing before the interruption.

One thing that helps is to be very aware of the context switch. I guess we could call that "lucid switching." You tell yourself, very consciously: "I'm now going to do *X*, then I will return to *Y*." It's like taking a mental picture. When the time comes to return to the original task, it will be easier to recall what that was.

Don't interrupt an interruption

It becomes more difficult when you stack interruptions. When dealing with an interruption, you should not allow another interruption because switching back then becomes much more difficult. You might forget the original task (might?) and coming back to it will often take so much longer.

If the second interruption can somehow be averted or delegated, do so. If a colleague is asking you to take a look at an issue or to have a meeting, you may request to send an email or to ask you again in an hour. If it's a child, you may promise to talk to it as soon as you're finished with what you were doing.

When there's no alternative

But of course things aren't always so clear-cut. When you can't avert or delegate the new interruption, see if you can delegate what you were doing, and make a note somehow of what you have to return to later. A technique I sometimes use, when I have to context-switch and don't have much time, is to write a quick note to myself and stick it where I will definitely notice it. Another is to write myself a quick telegram-style email. Email is something I check very regularly during the day, and so I'm bound to pick up where I left off soon.

Avoid Morning Stress

When you start your day stressfully, this will have an impact on the rest of your day. Rushing through the morning routine, skipping breakfast or having a bit in your car, then cursing through the traffic hardly begets a good, productive day.

Still, stressful mornings seem more the rule than the exception nowadays, especially for the night owls among us. We prefer to stay in bed as long as we can and then race through the motions to get ready for work. Then on the road we remember all the things we forgot to do or bring, and we notice we are wearing spotted or wrinkled clothes. If, on top of it all, we have children to take care of, this part of the day can really stress us out.

Stress causes our body to produce so-called "stress hormones", such as cortisol and norepinephrine. These increase heart rate and thus blood pressure. Norepinephrine, which also transmits fight-or-flight response signals throughout the body, is believed to play a role in hypertension, depression and ADD. You don't want that baby to fire up unless it has to.

Here are some tips to take the edge off the mornings.

Rise 15 minutes early

What? Yes. We like to catch as many *Zzzs* as we can, but time is an important factor in the morning stress equation. If we calculate the exact time we need to leave before traffic hits, and then (under-) estimate the time needed for breakfast, showering and getting dressed, we cannot afford anything to go wrong in the morning routine. You check your clothing and find that your shirt is spotted? Now you'll have to waste valuable minutes changing.

But if you built in, say, 10 minutes of *contingency time* to allow for such intrusions, and leave the house five minutes earlier so that at least the trip to work or school will be a bit less stressful, wouldn't that save a lot of headaches and anxiety? Would it not give you more peace of mind to know that, yes, even though traffic is its usual charming self, it has less impact on your schedule? Surely that must be worth 15 minutes of sleep?

Of course the 15 minutes I'm talking about here is an example; your mileage may vary. Maybe 10 or 20 minutes will work better for you, but you get the idea.

Prepare your morning

A little preparation the night before saves time and hassle in the morning. Preselect (and check) your clothes, set the breakfast table and prepare the kids' school bags. Not only will the next morning be less hectic, you might actually sleep better knowing you're prepared. See also the next chapter, "Establish a Bedtime Ritual".

No breakfast TV

I'm not trying to sound like a strict stepmother, but TV in the morning does not help. Watching TV while you're having breakfast is not only unhealthy, it also takes more time and does not promote family bonding. Just leave the TV off; you'll catch the news later.

Use a morning checklist

Here's another one of those checklists. A morning checklist provides a good guideline for establishing and checking your morning routine and for making sure you don't forget anything. If, when you leave the house, everything on the checklist is crossed off, you will be more at ease the rest of the day. If there are still items on the list, at least you know.

I have a fixed checklist that I know by heart by now, but I still go over it every morning. Sometimes I'll add or remove items as necessary, but the list has been fairly static for the last few months. It keeps me from forgetting or skipping tasks and feeling bad about it afterwards.

For more about planning your day, and improving how you handle work vs. time, check out *http://www.daytimer.com*. The site also has tips on how to handle interruptions, how to plan for calls, and so forth.

Establish a Bedtime Ritual

It's very important to establish a routine, or ritual, to end the day serenely. We need to get our brains into "peace and quiet" mode before we go to bed, so that we can enjoy a good night's sleep. According to WebMD, some 35% of Americans suffer from insomnia. And getting a good night's rest is even more important to us ADDers than "regular" people. Our brains don't have an *Off* button, so we need to get them to a state as close as possible. So it's a good thing we are creatures of habit, because this enables us to get into a helpful routine quickly.

But the whole process of going to sleep, and getting your brain into sleep mode, is highly complex and very individual. You need to figure out what works for you. For me, reading is a good way to cut off my brain's train of thought and doze off, but for you it may do the opposite.

No news right before bed – better yet, no TV

It's a scientific fact that watching TV is an ADD trigger in children. A study from the American Academy of Pediatrics indicated that watching TV as a toddler may lead to ADD. This is related to the high pace of TV programs and movies, which doesn't match real life. If you compare TV shows of the 2000's to those of, say, the 1970s, it becomes clear that the action is much speedier, the cutting more aggressive. According to the study, this overstimulates toddlers' brains, which causes permanent changes in the connections made in the brain. TV is one of the things that get our brains into racing mode.

It should be no surprise to us that if we want to get our heads to wind down, we should be careful what we watch right before bed, if anything at all. This means no news, no sports, or anything that gets our mind to pay attention.

My bedtime ritual used to include watching the news right before flicking off the TV. This was a bad habit because some of those images just kept on replaying in my head during the night. Since I dropped watching news so late, I sleep a lot better.

Whether you need to drop TV altogether, say, ½ hour before you go to sleep, is something you'll need to figure out on your own. This rule does work for me, but your mileage may vary. Sleep is a very complicated issue, and you may find a different strategy more beneficial. If you're struggling with insomnia, see a doctor.

Here are some other tactics you may find useful:

Take a warm bath

A warm bath relaxes your muscles and gets your mind off things. Pour a relaxing oil or foam in the water. Scented candles and soft music help set the mood for a quiet, peaceful night.

Special relaxation CD's and white noise CD's are available everywhere music is sold. Take some time out and drift away. If you want to limit your bathing time to, say, 30 minutes, then put the music on an MP3 player or phone and let it play for that period. You'll know time is up when the music stops.

White noise

Some people need white noise, like a hum, to catch sleep. It may help to spend the last ½ hour of the day doing laundry just for that reason. Maybe your partner can drive around while you rest in the back seat of the car. The feeling of driving and the repetitive sound of the engine may just do the trick.

Only light snacks right before bedtime

If you're hungry but it's (almost) bedtime, it's OK to have a snack as long as it's light. The digestive system slows down while you sleep, so rich snacks can cause problems such as reflux. According to WebMD, it's best not to eat a heavy meal within *four hours* of going to bed.

For a bedtime snack, a small bowl of cereals with milk or a few cookies are good choices: rich in carbohydrates and not too much hard-to-digest protein.

Hot milk

Drink hot milk or hot cocoa. Hot milk helps you doze off; it's a scientific fact. Milk contains two ingredients that help you relax (calcium and L-tryptophan), and chocolate adds to the sensation of well-being, thanks to the anandamide it contains. Alternatively, you may try linden tea or valerian root tea, both of which induce sleep.

When do you take your last ADD meds?

Do your meds keep you up at night? Some of us, research suggests, sleep *better* when under the influence of stimulant medication, whereas others – myself included – have difficulty getting to sleep. If you are in the latter category too, experiment with the latest hour you can take your meds before they start keeping you up at night. For me, it means I cannot take my Ritalin after 4 PM as a general rule. Of course many factors influence sleep patterns, such as how tense you are and whether you've slept well the last few days. But make sure you know approximately when it's too late to take any more medication.

An example bedtime routine

Here's my current bedtime routine. I call the time I actually go to bed "T". This time "T" varies per day, but is usually around 11:30 PM.

- T minus 4 hours: No more heavy meals.

- T minus 30 minutes: No more TV, PC. I check my phone's battery, and may charge it during the last 30 minutes of the day.
  - I spend this time reading, or relaxing on the couch with music, or just "doing nothing".
  - I check my phone's morning alarm to make sure I'll wake up at the right time.
- T minus 10 minutes: If I have to get up really early, I prepare the table for breakfast (usually just cereal, so that is easy to do, but it feels good that the table is set when I come downstairs in the morning).
- T minus 5 minutes: I go upstairs to brush my teeth and get undressed.
- T: I go to bed.

Power Naps are Good for You

Don't be afraid of napping during daytime, unless it keeps you from sleeping at night. If you can nap after lunch for, say, 20 to 30 minutes, then you'll be more alert in the afternoon. Again, scientific research has shown that napping enhances the brain's information processing and learning abilities.

From a NIMH press release (July 2, 2002):

New experiments by NIMH grantee Alan Hobson, M.D., Robert Stickgold, Ph.D., and colleagues at Harvard University show that a midday snooze reverses information overload and that a 20 percent overnight improvement in learning a motor skill is largely traceable to a late stage of sleep that some early risers might be missing. [...]

The bottom line: we should stop feeling guilty about taking that "power nap" at work or catching those extra winks the night before our piano recital.

Of course, it's not always easy to close your eyes during the daytime. Your work situation may not allow it. But if you go to work by car, maybe you can slip into your car over lunch and nap a little there.

Prepare For Important Conversations

If you have an important meeting scheduled, or even if you need to make a phone call, it pays tremendously to spend a few minutes preparing.

Go over the conversation in your mind, and make notes. Say that you need to call a painter, to ask for a cost estimate to paint your house. The painter will have to see your house, so you'll need to make an appointment. Maybe your spouse can let the painter in; then you won't have to be there. But you may *want* to be there, to give specifics. When would be a convenient time? Do you prefer to do this during the week or over the weekend, in the morning or in the afternoon? How urgent is the paint job? What is your budget?

All of these questions come to mind, and it's best to think about them *before* placing the call. So spend some time preparing, write down notes, and then call. The call will go easier when you understand what you need.

Bad news or difficult conversations

It is especially important to prepare for a conversation when you have to deliver bad news or when you expect the conversation to be difficult. Understand the essence and know how you're going to deliver the message. Keep in mind the person's situation and sensitivities.

If you fail to do this, and have to improvise, chances are you'll use the wrong words to convey the meaning.

Setting

For difficult conversations, you'll also want a proper setting – quiet and discreet, so that there are no distractions and you cannot be disturbed. When having such exchanges at home, turn off the TV, the radio and even the computer. Sit opposite your conversation partner and have no barriers in-between – such as notebooks, pots and pans, etc. Use notes if you must, to make sure you stay on track and you deliver your important message well.

Prepare for discussion

You may anticipate that your conversation partner will argue. Prepare for arguments. What do you expect him or her to say? Are those arguments valid? If not, why not? Preparing well means that you'll be far less distracted by details during the discussion, and that improves the chances of a beneficial outcome.

The Monday Morning Rule

On Monday morning, many of us are still slowly awaking from the weekend, getting ready for the rest of the week. So as a rule, try to avoid difficult or very important meetings on Monday mornings. It's best to discuss things when everyone has full access to their wits.

Time and Attention Magnets Lead to Compulsion

We get distracted easily, that's no big news. So if we want to be on time more often, be in full possession of our faculties more often, and generally lower our stress levels, we should recognize what is most distracting to us, and discard those distractions.

Time and attention magnets can lead to addiction and compulsion, two of the biggest enemies of ADDers. Addiction and compulsion, in turn, lead to all kinds of problems, including sleep deprivation and chronic procrastination. What follows now is a non-exhaustive list of these time and attention magnets, which we should avoid.

"Social" networks

Prime examples are mostly useless diversions such as **Facebook** and **Twitter**. People get hooked on those, but, honestly, what do they really add to our lives? How many really interesting tweets have you read lately? Do you care what your friend is having for breakfast, or that during his latest trip out of town he had an epiphany about boy bands (and they were *a-rockin'*)? Do you truly think that if you join Facebook you'll have 200 "friends"?

I know many people that are on Twitter and Facebook, and when I ask them what they get out of it, almost always they murmur something like "it's something to do", or "my friends are on it, so..." They spend hours online and they get distracted every time someone tweets even the most irrelevant tidbit.

I'm not trying to be the party-pooper here, but how bad is that for us, the easily distracted? Having accounts on "social" services like

Twitter and Facebook is mostly a waste of time, and quite the opposite of what we need. If you absolutely want to be social, join a discussion group or a sports club – they are actually good for your social skills.

Furthermore, there is scientific evidence that social networks have a negative impact on users' attention span and sense of reality. Prof. Greenfield, specializing in synaptic pharmacology at Lincoln College, Oxford (U.K.) warns that experiences on social networking sites "are devoid of cohesive narrative and long-term significance. As a consequence, the mid-21st century mind might almost be infantilized, characterized by short attention spans, sensationalism, inability to empathize and a shaky sense of identity." She adds, "It might be helpful to investigate whether the near total submersion of our culture in screen technologies over the last decade might in some way be linked to the threefold increase over this period in prescriptions for methylphenidate, the drug prescribed for attention-deficit hyperactivity disorder."

In short: social networking exacerbates ADD.

See also "How to Quit Facebook" at *http://www.wikihow.com/Quit-Facebook*.

Video gaming

Another common black hole for time is video gaming. I know quite a few compulsive gamers, and the more they play, the more it seems to consume them. Even at family gatherings or their own birthday parties, they play online games on a computer or on a hand-held device. When you ask them to direct their attention to the conversation or the people around them, they get cranky. Video games are, in a way, an escape hatch from social anxiety. Like social network sites, online video games provide a seemingly safe way to interact with others without actually having to face them. It is especially when games are used as an escape, that gaming leads to addiction and compulsion, and can take over a person's life.

The aforementioned Prof. Greenfield states in her research, when discussing video games, "The sheer compulsion of reliable and almost immediate reward is being linked to similar chemical systems in the brain that may also play a part in drug addiction. So we should not underestimate the 'pleasure' of interacting with a screen when we puzzle over why it seems so appealing to young people."

For more information and to get counseling, see *http://www.video-game-addiction.org*.

Compulsive gambling

Science has also linked ADD to compulsive gambling. Research has indicated that people who gamble compulsively, or who are addicted to gambling or gambling-like activities such as online poker, have genetic disorders that block dopamine receptors in the brain. Studies have shown that some 20% of people diagnosed with compulsive gambling also have ADD, and some 35% have other impulsive disorders.

A problem with gambling is easy to recognize: if it obstructs your life – for example, if you miss meetings or you are perpetually tired because you play online poker well into the night – then it is a problem and must be handled. I used to play poker online, and played well from 11 PM until 2 AM or even later, sometimes even until the time I would have had to get up to go to work. I lost far too much sleep and became very irritable and even aggressive. I could not handle it when I lost from a player whose ability was obviously inferior to mine, only because he got lucky. I have even damaged my desk because I "hit the roof" when I lost, in the middle of the night, awakening my spouse and probably my neighbors. Online poker had become a problem for me rather than a pastime.

The only way to deal with this problem is to get or stay away from it. This is especially difficult if you live alone, because there is less social control and peer pressure to keep you away from the gaming tables. But if you have a partner, enlist his or her help.

Stay away from casinos, including online casinos. Turn off your PC at least ½ hour before you go to bed (see also the chapter on establishing sleep rituals). Even if your habit is mildly profitable, as was my online poker habit, it's something to let go if it swallows too much of your time and if it makes you irritable or distracted.

For more information and to get counseling, see *http://helpguide.org/mental/gambling_addiction.htm.*

Other distractions

Identify what distracts you. Is your desk quite clean but you keep looking at that great picture of your dog? Maybe it's better to put the picture somewhere else, so that you can focus on work while behind the desk. Do you get distracted by the sports bar you drive by on the way to work? Maybe it would help to take a different route. If the tick-tock-tick-tock of the wall clock drives you crazy, throw it out and get a silent clock.

Look around you and see what your time and attention magnets are, and find a way around them. You'll become a calmer person.

Build a Support System

Building a support system is one of the most important things a person with ADD must do. You cannot do it all alone. It's an exhausting, confusing world out there, and everyone can use a little help. Add our inherent chaos to the mix and it's easy to see that help is essential for us. It's just something we need. There is no shame in asking for help, and we have lots to give in return.

Tell your family

It's important to let your immediate family know about your ADD. Your family probably knows you more intimately than anyone else. Tell them what you discovered, and how you discovered it. It will make sense to them, just like it made sense to you. They too will feel the relief of that missing puzzle piece falling into place. They will remember situations and suddenly understand what was really going on. So *that* was why you did what you did and said what you said?

To help them understand better, you may have to educate them about what it is like, being you. Explain to them that there are some things you excel at, and other things you need help with. Buy them a book on adult ADD if you have to.

Your family, and certainly your spouse, is your first Support line, the one you need the most.

Discussion groups

You may also join an Adult ADD discussion group. There are plenty of ADD forums on the Internet, but it is much better to join an actual, living, breathing, "live" discussion group in your area. It helps to be able to talk to fellow ADDers and hear that they struggle with the exact same things you struggle with. Some may have come up with solutions that you never thought of (just like the strategies in this book). When I first went to an adult ADD discussion night, I felt so relieved! Suddenly I had many people to talk to who knew exactly what I was going through, who could relate. Nothing compares to that.

Often these discussion groups meet once or twice per month. There is usually a discussion theme to every meeting. For example, there may be meetings about relationships, to which you can bring your partner. This is an excellent opportunity to show, rather than tell, your partner about the world that ADDers live in. Visit CHADD at *http://www.chadd.org* for discussion groups in your area.

Exercise and Diet partners

If you have difficulty exercising – or rather, getting to it –, get an exercise partner. Go to the gym together, play tennis together, or any sport that you both like. It is not only much more fun to do activities together, it also creates a soft sort of peer pressure to keep up the exercise. It is also a mental boost not to have to do this alone.

By the same token, if you need to diet, it's important to have a diet partner. Ideally your spouse becomes your diet partner, which automatically sets constraints on available foods. It also helps if you don't have to watch your spouse empty a bag of potato chips while you have just a glass of water.

It is generally a good idea, when dieting, to join a group such as Weight Watchers. You can go to the meetings regularly (say once per week), weigh yourself, keep a weight log and mingle with fellow dieters. This gives a boost to your diet and helps you to keep on track.

Friends and colleagues

You may have friends and colleagues who share your condition. Have you talked to them about it yet? In my career I have often brought up the subject of ADD to coworkers; mostly coworkers I suspected of being "members of the club". In some cases, this led to *aha*-moments in those coworkers' minds, and they went and got themselves diagnosed!

It's good to have people close to you who understand ADD. If you have friends and coworkers who have it too, you can support each other. For instance, you may help each other to get tasks done on time, even if all your friend needs is a timekeeper or a reviewer. Sometimes you just need to bounce some ideas or thoughts off of a colleague who can relate. Talk about it and help each other out.

The right person for the right job

One of my mottos in life is: "Give the job to the person who is competent to do it". That extends itself to all aspects of life. I'm terrible at plumbing, so I delegate that task to someone who is good at it. I'm also terrible with opening paper mail and following up, so I enlist the help of my wife who excels at it. As a final example, I never file my own tax returns; I hire an accountant to do that. It costs some money, sure, but not filing tax returns on time, or filing faulty returns costs more.

You have lots to give in return

Remember that when you get help from others, it's only natural that you return the favor. While your neighbor may be good at painting, maybe you can fix his computer or help his teenager with math. Be creative in how you return the favor. We may need lots of help but, just like everyone else, there are many things we are good at.

BONUS SECTION: 4 x 10

This bonus section's chapters are different from the rest of the book.

They are all Lists of 10:

- 10 Reasons to invest in a smartphone
- 10 Books to Read
- 10 Websites to Explore
- 10 Blogs about ADD

So we end the book with a set of lists rather than chapters with practical tips. Most of these are also longer than the other chapters in the book.

10 Reasons to Invest in a Smartphone

Today's smartphones are just about the handiest devices on the planet. And you don't even need ADD to appreciate the level of organization these machines can bring to your life. Seriously, a modern smartphone is an absolute must-have. Once you get one, you'll be hooked (but as always, know when to put it down and enjoy your *real* life).

Here are 10 things to look for when deciding what smartphone to buy:

1. A good phone

Of course we all need a good telephone. You want a device with good, clear reception. It should have a decent battery life, so that you don't need to charge it every four hours.

2. A high-speed Internet connection and WiFi

Any self-respecting smartphone nowadays has support for 3G or 4G Internet and Wi-Fi (local wireless), and a built-in Web browser. With an always-on Internet connection, you really have "information at your fingertips", as Bill Gates so prophetically expressed it back in 1990.

3. Automated calendar

This is also essential. If you want to organize your meetings, appointments, dates and the like, you really need an automated calendar. What's more, you need a *single* calendar that you can use from different sources such as your PC and your phone. Therefore, you need a phone that comes with properly integrated automatic calendaring.

With such software, you can type in appointments with full details such as date and time, location, and who else is invited. You can get a reminder at a time of your convenience, and your smartphone can even give you an overview of all upcoming appointments, or a weekly or monthly overview. You'll never forget a doctor's appointment again! It's so effortless that it borders on criminal not to use it.

Personally, I use Google Calendar. Other possibilities are Microsoft's Windows Live Calendar or Outlook, Bravenet, Cozi, etc. There are many options, but I use Google Calendar because it is feature-rich, free, and available everywhere. I can enter an appointment on my PC and it's visible immediately on my phone, and vice versa. I can invite my wife to events (she also has a smartphone with Google Calendar on it), and we can coordinate our schedules with ease.

Related to the calendar is the "alarm clock" feature found on all smartphones. I have a set of weekday alarms set up: one for waking up with classical music, one to sternly warn me I have to leave for work in 10 minutes, one right before lunchtime and another one to warn me I have to leave work within minutes, or miss my train home. A simple feature like this can make a big difference.

4. E-mail

Another obvious must-have is e-mail support. A good phone can organize multiple e-mail-addresses. You can download and read your e-mails in real time, you can write e-mails and save drafts, attach files, you name it.

5. Camera

A nice camera goes a long way. Even when you forgot your expensive camera at home, you can take decent pictures. Certainly the new devices that are hitting the market nowadays come with excellent cameras. Make sure yours includes a LED flash.

If your phone can also record video, so much the better. You can "tape" unexpected events such as the little one's first steps, or record evidence when you become an accidental witness. And why not take a picture of your car when you park it somewhere, to serve as a reminder later?

When you take the family out to crowded places such as amusement parks or markets, quickly take two pictures of your kids: one close-up and one full. In the unfortunate case that you lose track of one of them, you can show police or bystanders *exactly* what they look like, rather than relying on a studio picture taken six months before.

A friend of mine used his phone's video camera feature in a creative and interesting way. He went to purchase something in a store and the salesman on duty was less than friendly. My friend took out his phone, started to record a video and asked, "Would you please repeat that?"

6. GPS

Built-in GPS is just great. Even when you have no clue where you are, just open that Map application and you know. If your phone supports extended Map applications such as Google Maps or Bing Maps, you can even look up the nearest gas station, hotel, school, restaurant, police station, or whatever you are looking for.

A nice side-use of built-in GPS with a Maps application is that you can use it to tag the location of your car. Just put a "pin" on your present location on the map when you leave the car, and at the end of the day you won't have to comb out the neighborhood to retrieve your ride.

7. Music and video player

Why carry around an MP3 player or other media device with you, when your phone will do just fine? I haven't touched my 8GB MP3 player since I got a decent phone (with a 16GB SD memory card). To top it off, the media player in my phone can do all sorts of neat tricks with my music, such as slow it down without altering pitch, etc.

It's also nice when you can view video files. When stuck in a huge jam when there was an accident on the freeway, I recently took out my phone and watched an episode of *Friends* that I had converted to MP4 format earlier. Out went the stress.

8. Integrated search

Integrated search is a way of finding information or files on your phone and/or the Internet. You can locate music files, pictures, Word documents, PDF documents etc. that are stored on your phone, or you can look for similar images on the Web etc.

With smart applications such as Google Voice Search, you can even dictate what you're looking for and the phone will find it on the Web. With another application, Google Goggles, you can take a picture and have the application look for similar pictures (and thus identify what you took a picture of) on the Web.

Another fun application that modern phones have is barcode scanning. Using your phone's camera, you can "scan" a barcode such as a regular EAN code used on food packaging, but also QR codes used on packages, in advertisements, etc. You can thus search for information just by scanning a barcode.

9. Airplane Mode (automated, please)

Airplane Mode is a feature of phones where you turn off communications, but can still use the other features of the phone. Its name is of course derived from the fact that you are not allowed to keep your phone turned on on an airplane, as it can interfere with communications systems.

I have an application on my phone that automatically switches the phone to Airplane Mode at 11 PM, if I'm not making a call. Then in the morning at 7:45, it automatically switches Airplane Mode off again. I never have to think of switching my phone on or off.

10. Downloadable software

And this brings us to our final point: downloadable software. For all currently popular smartphone systems – Android, Windows Mobile, iPhone and BlackBerry – there are online marketplaces where you can instantly download thousands of applications for free or for a very low price.

Some of these applications are very basic and have only one function – such as helping you find back your car, or automatically turning Airplane Mode on and off, or using your camera's LED light as a flashlight. Other applications are very extensive, for example word processors and spreadsheets.

With downloadable applications, you can keep extending and customizing your phone to really fit your needs.

10 Books to Read

I recommend the following books:

1. Is it You, Me, or Adult A.D.D.?

Pera, Gina, 2008. *Is it You, Me, or Adult A.D.D.?* 1201 Alarm Press. Available in paperback and PDF editions. A good, thorough (and thus long) treatise on all aspects of adult ADD, mostly with regard to relationships and unrecognized/untreated ADD. This is probably one of the most comprehensive non-clinical works on the subject. It is the only consumer's book that explains what kind of therapy is recommended for ADHD (CBT for ADHD) – and in detail. It is the only non-clinical book to detail the medication protocol (which is so important, and so overlooked by 90% of physicians.)

2. 10 Simple Solutions to Adult ADD

Sarkis, Stephanie, 2006. *10 Simple Solutions to Adult ADD: How to Overcome Chronic Distraction & Accomplish Your Goals.* New Harbinger Publications. Available in paperback and Kindle editions. Like the book you're reading now, Dr. Sarkis' book takes a rather practical approach to dealing with adult ADD.

3. Delivered From Distraction

Hallowell, Edward M., and Ratey, John J., 2005. *Delivered From Distraction.* Ballantine Books. Available in a multitude of formats. A very interesting discussion about the current body of knowledge about adult ADHD. The book also discusses how, to be successful, you must structure your life to minimize the impact of your weaknesses and to maximize your strengths. Both authors are not only psychiatrists and ADD experts, but are ADDers themselves as well.

4. Don't Sweat The Small Stuff

Carlson, Richard, 1996. *Don't Sweat The Small Stuff.* Hyperion. Available in hardcover, paperback, audio and Kindle editions. One hundred short musings on living life in a more relaxed and easy-going manner. Not only for ADD types, this book is a great resource to keep re-reading as it puts a lot of things in perspective.

5. End Procrastination Now!

Knaus, William, 2010. *End Procrastination Now!* McGraw-Hill. Available in paperback and Kindle editions. An interesting text about, guess what, procrastination and how to put a halt to it. It shows that procrastination is really an expression of fear, and that "later" is most often not "better." On the downside, it's lengthy – the paperback version is 256 pages.

6. It's All Too Much

Walsh, Peter, 2007. *It's All Too Much: An Easy Plan for Living a Richer Life with Less Stuff*. Free Press. Available in a multitude for formats. This book is not targeted only at ADD folk, but to all whose lives can use better organization and less hoarding.

7. Taking Charge of Adult ADHD

Barkley, Russell A, 2010. *Taking Charge of Adult ADHD*. The Guilford Press. Available in hardcover, paperback and DRM-protected PDF (on eBooks.com). A very impressive volume, this book will probably become the classic ADD book for patients as well as healthcare professionals. Barkley treats the disorder from A to Z including medications and their (side-) effects, non-medical treatments, tips and tricks, and the myth that ADHD is a "gift". This is another lengthy volume, at almost 300 pages.

8. The Checklist Manifesto

Awande, Atul, 2009. *The Checklist Manifesto: How to Get Things Right*. Metropolitan Books. Available in hardcover, paperback, audio and Kindle editions. Dr. Awande illustrates, from his perspective as a surgeon, how to organize work and how to get results and a personal sense of satisfaction. Obviously, using checklists is a key ingredient.

9. Time Management In An Instant

Leland, Karen and Bailey, Keith, 2008. *Time Management In An Instant: 60 Ways to Make the Most of Your Day.* Career Press. Available in paperback and Kindle editions. An easy to chew book which covers 60 varied tips on time management in just 160 pages.

10. What Causes ADHD?

Nigg, Joel T, 2009. *What Causes ADHD?* The Guilford Press. Available in hardcover, paperback and DRM-protected PDF (on eBooks.com). This clinical volume treats the causes of ADHD in children, explaining what influences young children's brains and how. Not for the faint of heart, but if you really want to know how it "clicks" then this is the book to wrestle through.

10 Websites to Explore

I recommend the following websites to explore. You can find these and many more in the *Links* section of this book's website, *http://www.addsimplified.com*.

1. About ADD

A general, and very rich, resource on ADD with medical and psychological information, links to ADD-related websites and articles. This is a good first stop to point people to who want to learn about ADD.

http://add.about.com

2. ADDA – Attention Deficit Disorder Association

The official website of the (U.S.) Attention Deficit Disorder Association.

http://www.adda.org

3. ADD Forums

Online forums about all topics related to ADD, including ADD at work, in relationships, parenting, and similar conditions such as Asperger's Syndrome and Learning Disabilities.

http://www.addforums.com

4. ADDitude Magazine

The official website of ADDitude Magazine; as it name suggests, a periodical about life as an ADDer.

http://www.additudemag.com

5. ADDvance

An extensive resource on all aspects of ADD, including parenting, education, workplace issues, women's issues and the like. This site started out focusing on women's issues with relation to ADD, but has since expanded its scope to a wider audience.

http://www.addvance.com

6. ADHD Europe

An extensive resource for European AD(H)D healthcare professionals as well as patients.

http://www.adhdeurope.eu/home.html

7. ADHD News

General resource about ADHD, with links to medical and diet information, books and websites.

http://adhdnews.com

8. ADHD Rollercoaster

The companion website to Gina Pera's book *Is It You, Me or Adult A.D.D.?* You can read a chapter of this book online, and join the publisher's mailing list.

http://www.adhdrollercoaster.com

9. CHADD

The official websites of **Children and Adults with Attention-Deficit Disorder,** a nonprofit organization providing education, advocacy and support for persons with AD(H)D. CHADD publishes **Attention Magazine**.

http://www.chadd.org

10. Organized Wisdom: ADHD

This site is mostly a collection of links, fast facts etc., nicely categorized, about all health issues.

http://www.organizedwisdom.com/adhd

10 Blogs about ADD

The blogosphere is buzzing with ADD-related blogs. Here are some I visited recently and found particularly interesting. I find it striking that, while adult ADD is primarily associated with men (the ratio is estimated to be 3:1), most of these blogs are written by women.

1. Jeff's ADD Mind

The blog, with audio and even video podcasts, of the ever-lucid Jeff Siegel. Jeff rants on-camera and on the microphone with razor-sharp observations and enlightening discourse about all matters ADD.

http://www.jeffsaddmind.com

2. You and Me – and Adult AD/HD

Another site from Gina Pera, expert by experience and author. She adds another post every first Tuesday of the month.This blog used to focus on the relationship aspects of ADD, but now covers life with ADD in a broader sense.

http://adultadhdrelationships.blogspot.com

3. A Mom's View of ADHD

What's it like to be the mother of a child with ADD/ADHD? In other words, what did our mothers have to go through when we were young, and what are the worries, traps and delights mothers with ADHD children are facing today? Their perspective, and their insights, apply to us adult ADDers as well.

http://adhdmomma.blogspot.com

4. Mungo's Adult Attention Deficit Hyperactivity Disorder

Musings of an adult father with ADHD, well written and touching. I particularly like his journal of how he tried out Strattera, and his beautiful pictures of nature.

http://www.mungosadhd.com

5. Primarily Inattentive ADD

This is the blog of Tessermom, a mother of two sons with the syndrome, and a "member of the in-crowd" herself. Tessermom discusses things like food supplements, different types of treatment, and scientific research.

http://www.primarilyinattentiveadd.com

6. My ADD / ADHD Blog

ADD/ADHD Coach Tara McGillicuddy. She blogs about various aspects, including whether the name "ADHD" is in fact correct (a topic that Gina Pera also touches upon), the daily struggles that come with our "gift", upcoming conferences, support groups etc.

http://www.myaddblog.com

7. Stephanie Sarkis

This site is the Web home of Dr. Stephanie Sarkis, author of books such as 10 Simple Solutions to Adult ADD and ADD And Your Money. Dr. Sarkis regularly updates her blog and talks about various issues such as medication, food allergies, ADHD children's fears, etc. The site also features some podcasts and radio interviews.

http://www.stephaniesarkis.com/blog

8. New Ideas.Net

The blog of Dr. Douglas Cowan, although the title doesn't suggest it, focuses on ADD/ADHD. One of the main topics of this blog is alternative ADHD treatments, i.e. without stimulant medication.

http://newideas.net

9. ADHD from A to Zoë

The blog of Zoë Kessler, a woman who struggles with ADHD (and very specifically the Hyperkinetic part). A professional writer who got her diagnose at 47, Zoë writes about all aspects of ADHD, including the impact on her own life.

http://blogs.psychcentral.com/adhd-zoe

10. ADHD.tv

The video podcast of Dr. Kenny Handelman, ADHD.tv is a collection of YouTube-posted videos on mostly the diagnostic and treatment side of ADD/ADHD.

http://www.adhd.tv

Final Thoughts

We're at the end of this book. So far I have nothing more to share. I hope you enjoyed it, and that you'll often come back to it. It's been a great ride for me and I'm sure that the companion website will extend that ride for all of us.

A word of caution, though. No amount of strategies, tactics, tips and tricks will ever replace medication and counseling. The strategies outlined in this book help you to deal with the effects of our common syndrome, but there is no substitute for proper, optimized-for-you medication and professional help. Rather, these strategies are complementary to medical and psychological treatment. They will definitely improve your life, but they'll never reach their potency unless you also take medication that works for you, and without regular counseling with a qualified professional.

If you'd like to share your story, or a golden tip, or if you'd just like to see what others have shared, come to the site, *http://www.addsimplified.com*. See you there!

Sincerely,

Sidney Parker Holt

November 2010

ADD Simplified, Other Editions

This book is available in the following editions:

Kindle. Available only on Amazon, at $9.95 and Amazon UK, at £ 7.18.

ISBN-13: 978-0-9831511-0-4

Nook. Available only at Barnes & Noble, at $9.95.

ISBN-13: 978-0-9831511-2-8

EPUB. For the iPad, iPhone, and Sony Reader. Available at the Apple iBookstore and the Sony Reader Store, at $9.99.

ISBN-13: 978-0-9831511-2-8

Paperback. Available at Amazon and many other retailers at $14.95.

ISBN-13: 978-0-9831511-1-1

We may also publish an audio version, if there is enough interest. If you'd like such a version, please let us know at *info@addsimplified.com*. Thank you!

Index

Airplane Mode (in smartphones), 110, 111
Android, 111
autopay, 54
Awande, Atul, 114
Bailey, Keith, 115
banks, 53
Barkley, Russell A, 114
bedtime ritual, 86, 89
Bing Maps, 109
BlackBerry, 111
books, 7, 22, 31, 39, 42, 43, 113, 118, 122
brain, 39, 41, 82, 89, 93, 99
budgeting, 53
cables, 19, 46, 47
calendar, 66, 69, 70, 75, 82, 107, 108
Carlson, Richard, 114
CHADD, 102, 118
Charron, Sylvain, 82
checklists, 21, 22, 23, 86
clothes, buying, 55
clutter, 27, 31, 35, 39, 49
color-coding, 13, 14, 15, 24
compulsion, 97, 98, 99
contingency time, 86
cortex, medial frontal, 82
coupons, 31, 32
credit cards, 57, 59, 61
curtains, 39
deadlines, 25, 66, 67
deadlines, self-imposed, 66
discussions, 96, 98, 101, 102, 113
distractions, 96, 97, 100

documents, 14, 27, 28, 39, 46, 47, 110
doorknob, 11
drawers, 14, 17, 18, 45, 46, 47
duality, 41
e-books, 8, 42, 43
electronics, 49, 75
e-mail, 15, 27, 28, 108
exercise, 102
Facebook, 97, 98
family, 13, 15, 18, 21, 53, 67, 86, 98, 101, 109
filing cabinets, 14, 27, 39, 41, 45, 46, 47
folders, 14
food, 18, 79, 110, 122
Fry, Prem, 79, 80
gambling, 54, 99, 100
gaming, video, 98
Google Calendar, 69, 108
Google Maps, 109
GPS, 76, 109
handbags, 37
impulse buying, 55
impulse control, 55
infomercials, 56
Internet, 28, 54, 76, 101, 107, 110
invoices, 27, 28, 54, 61
iPhone, 111
Kanban, 23, 24, 25, 82
keys, 11, 12, 13, 35, 36
Kindle, 42, 43, 113, 114, 115, 125
kitchen timers, 75
Knaus, William, 73, 114
Koechlin, Etienne, 82

labeling, 14, 17, 18, 45, 47

late, being, 12, 62, 69, 70, 71, 90, 91, 93

laundry, 49, 90

Leland, Karen, 115

Live Calendar, 108

Lost and Found, 47

luggage, 15

magazines, 31, 32, 42

magic marker, 18, 54

medication, 17, 46, 91, 114

milk, 18, 91

mirror, 11, 12, 55, 56

money, 31, 53, 54, 57, 59, 61, 67, 103, 122

mornings, 85, 96

newspapers, 42

Nigg, Joel T, 115

Outlook, 15, 75, 108

PDF files, 27, 110, 113, 114, 115

penalties and rewards, 67, 68, 73, 99

Pera, Gina, 113, 118, 121, 122

perfectionism, 79, 80

phone. See smartphone

pockets, 12, 36, 37, 61

power naps, 93

procrastination, 36, 65, 66, 68, 73, 79, 97, 114

relationships, 31, 79, 102, 113, 117

remembering, 11, 22, 36, 62, 65, 69, 85, 101

reminder, 11, 12, 69, 108, 109

robots, 49

Rule, Monday Morning, 96

Sarkis, Stephanie, 80, 113, 122

scanning, 15, 110

scissors, 35, 36, 37

shoes, 11, 31

showering, 75

Siegel, Jeff, 121

sleeping, 93

smartphone, 22, 66, 69, 75, 76, 105, 107, 108, 111

snacks, before bedtime, 91

spare change, 61

sticky notes, 22, 23, 24, 47

stress, 85

support, 15, 101, 103, 107, 108, 118, 122

tags, 27, 28

taxes, 14, 65, 67, 103

time management, 75, 115

toys, 14, 18, 31, 39, 42, 54

trays, 18

treasure chest, 39

tv, 19, 35, 56, 86, 89, 90, 92, 96

Twitter, 97, 98

wallet, 11, 12, 36, 61

Walsh, Peter, 114

watch, radio-controlled, 76

whiteboard, 22, 23

Windows Mobile, 111

www.ingramcontent.com/pod-product-compliance
Lightning Source LLC
Chambersburg PA
CBHW051738090426
42738CB00010B/2307